Guide to Couples love making
How to transform your sex life

Table of contents

Chapter 1

Understand the Difference Between Love-Making and Having sex

Many individuals often fail to see the differences between the two quite distinct activities of making love and having sex, whether they are men or women. Sex is an instinctual and bio-mechanical act that everyone can do, as stated on Thought Catalog. Making love, on the other hand, is seen as a sensuous, leisurely, and non-objective act that allows us the chance to feel the metaphysical being of oneness and is regarded as a kind of art in and of itself. As a result, little of each should be present in a healthy love relationship and satisfying sexual life.

Having sex versus making love

Sex or sexual activity, as seen on Teen Health Source, can mean different things to different people, but one thing is certain: most people find this to be a healthy and natural activity that they find meaningful in their particular ways. According to Austin Locke of Psychology Today, one may choose to commit this act for a variety of reasons, including lust, intimacy, boredom, relief, power play, expectation fulfillment, childbearing, expressing love, seeking comfort, etc. She continues by saying that this act is best understood as one of intimacy and sharing because there is no act more intimate than allowing another person access to a private body part to share pleasure.

Even though the phrases "having sex" and "making love" are frequently used interchangeably and even though making love frequently entails sexual activity, they do not always refer to the same thing.

When two people make love, their levels of vulnerability are quite high. As seen on Your

Tango, this frequently happens as a result of people sharing words and emotions that they may not have done before. Risk and reward are factors that come into play when both people tend to let their guard down. One feels particularly close to their partner while in a loving relationship and finds it difficult to imagine other moments happening without them.

On the other hand, although vulnerability still plays a part when you are having sex with someone, it takes a different form. In particular, one might worry that the sex won't be satisfying or lose the necessary chemistry. Another concern is whether or not one's sexual needs will be met, as described on Your Tango.

People who understand the difference also understand that, whether it involves the occasional missionary pose or more daring explorations, making love requires both parties to be completely themselves, genuine, and raw, like they are daily. Couples can completely relax and make love without feeling any pressure or restraint regarding their sexual needs or desires because of their shared love and understanding.

According to Your Tango, having sex does not always involve real feelings and emotions, and people sometimes allow themselves to be someone different than who they are normally. One can experiment with various sexual urges and reveal a side of themselves that they may never actually display in public. By engaging in sex, you might also be revealing some hidden personality traits.

Saying goodbye is never a problem and one may be able to move on without necessarily looking for commitment from the other side involved when love is not involved but only getting sexual pleasure. When you are having sex with someone you have a connection with, however, this is not always the case. Beyond receiving and giving sexual pleasure, making love involves sharing your feelings, emotions, and most private thoughts. Because of this, saying goodbye is not always simple, and both couples feel more devoted to one another.

As can be seen from the aforementioned observations, having sex and making love are two separate activities, with the former being more closely linked to receiving great physical pleasure via appropriate stimulation while the latter calls for receiving both sexual and romantic pleasure.

According to Thought Catalog, one need not be in love with the other person to have a great sexual encounter, and they may simply break up afterward. However, this is not the case when it comes to making love, which often necessitates exploring other areas, such as one's mind and soul, innermost emotions, and ideas, rather than simply each other's bodies. This leads to an increased degree of closeness and intimacy. Along with their love, the partners' passion often intensifies.

Having sex involves combining your bodily demands and body parts with the other partner, but making love mostly involves establishing a connection between your minds and souls via sexual activity.

Chapter 2

Benefit of Sexual Intimacy in Marriage and Relationship

Increasing sex in a supportive relationship has a lot of advantages. Positive changes like lower blood pressure, less stress, greater intimacy, and even a lower divorce rate are associated with higher rates of sexual activity. Sex in your relationship has advantages according to JR Bee's Verywell's illustration, Can a relationship last without sexual activity? Yes. Not always requires sex. However, it might play a significant role in a happy, healthy relationship.

Each person has a different perspective on the significance of sex. Some people might believe that having a sexual relationship is necessary. Others might believe that different forms of closeness and connection are more crucial.

You might believe that sex is significant in a relationship for the following reasons:

1. Being more intimate with your partner
2. Expressing love to your partner
3. Finding sex enjoyable
4. A desire to start a family
5. Feeling gorgeous and assured
6. Relieving stress According to research, regular sex may contribute to a person's overall wellbeing. More affection is frequently linked to having sex. Couples are more likely to have more frequent sex when they share more affection.

Although having sex less frequently does not automatically imply that your relationship is any less fulfilling, sex can be an important component of a relationship.

Benefits of Sexual Activity in Marriage

Regular sex has several benefits for a healthy relationship in addition to the advantages for you and your partner personally. For instance, the oxytocin produced during sex increases emotional intimacy and the sense of bonding.

Sex deepens your emotional connection and level of commitment to your partner in a monogamous relationship. Couples are more likely to remain together when they have sex to express their love. Sex is therefore positively linked to a lower divorce rate.

Benefits of Sex on the Mind

a. Makingve has numerous positive psychological and emotional effects (sex is strongly linked to a better quality of life). Among these advantages are:

a. Sexual activity can increase self-worth and lessen feelings of insecurity, which results in more positive perceptions of ourselves.

b. Higher levels of happiness: A 2015 Chinese study found that having more consensual sex and better-quality sex makes people happier.

c. More kinship Endorphins, one of the brain chemicals generated during sex, reduce irritation and depressive symptoms. The "hug drug," or another hormone, oxytocin, rises in response to nipple stimulation and other sexual activities. Oxytocin contributes to feelings of serenity and fulfillment.

d. Stress reduction: Less frequent sex may be attributed to chronic stress. However, having sex may be a useful stress-reduction strategy. The benefits of sexual activity linger long into the next day and lower stress response chemicals including cortisol and adrenaline (epinephrine).

e. Better sleep quality: Orgasms cause the release of the sleep-promoting hormone prolactin.

Physical Advantages of More Sex

Although it should be quite obvious how sex enhances mental wellness, there are also some physical advantages to having sex. A few of them are:

a. Improved physical fitness: Sex is an activity. Sexual engagement is similar to moderate physical exercise, such as brisk walking or ascending two flights of steps, according to the American Heart Association. Abdominal and pelvic muscles might become more toned and tightened during sex.

b. Improved muscular tone helps women have better bladder control.

c. Improved brain activity According to preliminary research on rats, more frequent sex sessions were associated with greater cognitive performance and the development of new brain cells. Since then, investigations on humans have shown similar advantages. In a 2018 research including over 6,000 people, regular sex was associated with superior memory function in those over the age of 50. Increased sexual activity has a good impact on immune system performance.

d. Regular sex may even reduce your risk of contracting the flu or a cold. lower degrees of discomfort Sexual endorphins contribute to more than only a calm and feeling of well-being. Additionally, it seems that sex endorphins lessen back and migraine discomfort.

e. Weight loss: A 30-minute session of sex typically burns 200 calories. Weight reduction may be assisted by the gratifying brain chemicals generated during sex, which can reduce cravings for food.

Positive Benefits on the Heart

a. Lower systolic blood pressure has been associated with penile-vaginal sexual activity, but not masturbation.

b. Heart disease and stroke risk are both increased by elevated blood pressure. By widening blood arteries, sexual activity lowers blood pressure and increases the flow of oxygen and nutrients throughout the body.

c. Additional physical advantages include an increase in desire and vaginal lubrication from increased sexual activity. Regular sexual activity is linked to shorter menstrual cycles and less uncomfortable cramps. In addition, the release of the hormone DHEA by the body during orgasm may be associated with an enhanced sense of smell, better teeth, better digestion, and radiant skin.

Ideal Sexual Frequency

A 2015 research indicated that, to a limited degree, sexual frequency is related to overall well-being when determining how often a couple should have sex. Relationship satisfaction increased gradually from no sex to once a week, but beyond that point, it stopped increasing (and even started to decline somewhat).

The present average is quite stable with one sexual interaction each week. However, our hectic schedules may be preventing us from engaging in more sex. Adults were having sex nine fewer times a year in 2010 than they were in the 1990s.

The typical sexual frequency, 54 times annually for the average adult (about once per week)
Adults in their twenties: Approximately 80 times yearly. Adults over 60: 20 times annually
Although frequency tends to decline with age, sexual activity is still significant in older persons. In general, older married couples engage in sexual activity more often than their single counterparts in the same age range.

Risks of Having More Sex

It was formerly thought that having intercourse made men more likely to get prostate cancer. However, a 2016 research found that males who ejaculated more often (21 or more times per month) were less likely to get the illness than those who ejaculated less frequently (seven or less per month). This impact is important to take note of since prostate cancer is the second biggest cause of cancer-related deaths in males.

For some people, having sex raises their risk of having a heart attack. Despite this danger, more frequent sex could be beneficial. According to 2011 research, frequent intercourse lowers the risk of heart attacks. Sex is protective, as are other physical activities. However, rare spurts of exercise put the heart under additional stress. To assess your risks, talk to your doctor about your sexual behavior.

The balance between the advantages and hazards may be tipped by unsafe sex. Make sure you are knowledgeable on safe sex procedures.

Problems with Regular Sex

While having sex might be crucial in a relationship, several things can make having sex more difficult. How often couples have sex may vary depending on several factors, including age, hormones, children, stress, illnesses, and marital issues.

Because sex hormone levels fall as individuals age, age often affects how frequently people have sex. Sometimes physical or psychological issues make having an active sex life difficult or impossible.The closeness of sex is what humans are designed to want. Lack of sex may cause partners to become distant and, perhaps, search for other partners. Working with a qualified couples therapist may help you close this gap and stop problems from affecting your whole marriage.

How to Develop Intimacy Without Sexual

By focusing on non-sexual techniques to increase closeness, couples may overcome these obstacles and continue to have a strong, healthy relationship. Consider the following ideas:

watching a movie or relaxing in the park while cuddling, dancing and engaging in other things you both like doing together. Giving plenty of kisses and hugs. Walking hand in hand while holding hands. Conversing often about How to Increase Sex in Your Relationship
Sexual activity may, and often does, fluctuate over time. However, this does not imply that sexual frequency must continue to decline unabated. The answer to the question of whether sex can still be as enjoyable as it was when you first fell in love is yes. With time and maturity in your

relationship, closeness and sex may grow. It could simply take a bit more effort.

There are several approaches to enliven your sexual life. It might be beneficial to consider your relationship's non-sexual aspects. The area between the ears is often referred to as the largest sex organ. Increased sex frequency without deeper emotional connection or better communication is unlikely to result in long-lasting relationship benefits. Another essential component of a healthy sexual life is stress management.

Throughout your relationship, you could modify how often you have sex. Your relationship may be strengthened and your sexual happiness can be increased by communicating with your spouse.

Getting Ready for a Sexy Night

A good relationship may benefit from having sexual activity. According to research, the typical American couple engages in sexual activity once a week. The frequency of sex tends to decrease with age, and other factors like stress, having kids, and general health may also have an impact. Sexual partners who wish to have more frequent encounters should concentrate on expressing their wants and cooperating.

Chapter 3

Conquer Your Shyness in the Bedroom.

Not all women can express their desires in the sex arena. You're just naturally shy about having sex, which is perfectly normal and doesn't indicate that you have a problem.

You may have frequently questioned why you felt awkward having sex with your husband.

Other questions that may come to mind in response to this one include "How can I stop being shy and awkward?" and "How can I please my husband in bed?"

You're not the only one who has this, and you can take action as well.

Don't believe that you can't get over your sexual shyness. You will feel more at ease during sexual activity if you have the right understanding and a mental shift.

Five causes of women's sexual shyness in bed

Women may be too shy for sex for a variety of reasons, even if it is with their spouse.

Some might believe that since you are already married, it is simpler to let go and be wild whenever you want to in bed. That isn't always the case, though. The majority of the time, shy wives still struggle to open up to their husbands.

There are a variety of reasons a woman might feel shy in bed, including:

1. You are timid by nature
"Why do I feel shy sexually with my husband" is a question that you may have

been thinking about for quite some time now. Deep inside, you know you also have sexual needs and wants, but what's stopping you? Some women are just naturally shy. For them, it's a challenge to be vocal about what they like and what they want.

2. You grew up in a conservative family
"That's not how a woman should behave." Some women grow up in a society where ladies are expected to be reserved and shy. Being too "open" about your sexuality or feeling sexually confident is perceived as being too vulgar and inappropriate in some communities or families. That's why even when married, some women become sexually awkward.

3. The media interprets "sexually confident" women differently
What's your first thought when you visualize yourself being wild in bed? "Sex makes me uncomfortable" may be one of the thoughts that will come to mind because when it

comes to women taking control of sex, you may visualize porn videos. You may even feel that it's not who you are, or you're not being yourself if you are in tune with your sexual desires.

4. You experience insecurity. Why do I feel awkward having sex with my husband? Is it a result of my outward appearance? Another typical explanation for why some women lack confidence in bed is this. We all struggle with insecurities, especially when we watch adult films and notice how attractive the actors are.

The idea of what a "sexy" woman should look like has been misrepresented by the film industry and even social media. Because of this, some women struggle with their sexual confidence.

5. You are concerned about your partner's opinion. "All I want is to keep my husband

content in bed, but I'm worried about what he might think," the wife confesses.

You desire to come out of your shell, be more assertive in bed, and act however you please, but you are afraid. You worry about what your husband will think of you. You fear that if something goes wrong, your marital bedtime chemistry may be jeopardized.

It's time to feel sexually confident now that you've addressed the causes of your reluctance to engage in sexual activity with your husband. You could improve your husband and wife relationship in the bedroom with these 8 straightforward tips. Some of these tips may even surprise you with how simple they are!

1 . Self-acceptance is important

It's time to let all of your restraints go. It's time to embrace who you are as the stunning and alluring woman that you are. We're telling you when you feel good about yourself, everything else will fall into place. Therefore, work on self-acceptance first before quitting being shy and awkward around your husband.

Let go and stop worrying about things that aren't that important. Your husband wants you, and you two are in this moment together.

2. Act on your behalf

You should decide to have sexual confidence. It's not out of concern that your husband might be unfaithful or because you feel under pressure from him to improve in bed. Act on your behalf. Decide because you want to and it will make you happy.

The next step is to be committed now that this is understood. To just let go and be wild won't be simple. If you make a sudden change, your spouse might be shocked. Being sexually confident requires time and commitment, just like any other kind of change.

3. Discover what makes you "on"
You must first ensure that you know yourself to be less shy and awkward with your husband concerning sexual matters. To be able to give pleasure, one must first be aware of their pleasures.

You must be aware of what makes you tick and what keeps you ticking. Love receiving sultry massages? Maybe a gentle kiss will turn you on. Never be afraid to ask for what you need. If you don't try it, how will you know? Do not be reluctant to compliment your husband on a job well done. If you want more, ask for it.

4. Invest in sexy attire

You won't know how good and sexy you will feel when you wear sexy clothes or lingerie until you have conquered any physical insecurities. Feeling sexy in what you're wearing is one of the benefits of having confidence in bed. Go ahead and surprise your husband by treating yourself to that lacey red underwear. Put on your preferred fragrance and turn down the lights.

5. Engage all of your senses

Knowing how to tickle your five senses can add spice to your sex life, given that we're already talking about setting the mood. Try scented candles, candy-flavored lube, plush feathers, sensual music, and, of course, blindfolds to get an idea. You'll experience increased sensuality and unforgettable love-making by engaging your senses. Not only will it give you exciting love life, but it will also make your marriage stronger.

6. Dare to assert yourself

Taking control can spice up your sex life, but you might want to discuss it with your husband first. Giving and receiving are the key to awesome sex life. Your husband might occasionally want to see you take the lead. So try it out without hesitation. Tie him up or perhaps blindfold him to gain control.

It's his turn to have his senses tricked this time. He won't be able to see what you're going to do to him, so you'll make him more aware of his other senses. It's unquestionably a fun treat for the two of you.

7. Entice and flirt

Do you think flirting is an art form? Being able to flirt requires courage, confidence, and sensuality because it involves sending subtle sexual cues. You simply can't get sex whenever you want it; you have to be able to create the right environment.

Give him a sensual massage or compose him a surprise letter, then tease him. Before he leaves for work, perhaps you could whisper something seductive? It can be fun and a great way to arouse sexual tension to learn how to flirt with your spouse.

8. Feel at ease doing what you're doing

Be at ease with what you are doing and love it. You'll not only get over your shyness in bed but you'll also be set free. Aside from that, you'll notice how much this can alter how your spouse and you perceive one another.

Stop being bashful in bed; your husband's sexual compatibility is crucial to your marriage. You'll become closer and feel more comfortable opening out to each other as a result. We are all aware of the positive effects that communication and closeness can have on a relationship. See how much it may improve your marriage by giving it your all.

Chapter 4

Use Sexting as Cue

Sexting may be scary, whether you're contacting someone you've been dating for a while or a stranger. We understand. But now is the perfect moment to start learning how to sext if you've been putting it off. Here is your comprehensive guide to sexting from experts.

1. Request permission

According to Mayour Craigh, licensed sex educator, just because you're ready to start sexting doesn't imply your sexting friend is. You must check in with your companion before you go from 0 to 60. Unless, of course, you've previously proved you have carte blanche for sexting, she argues.

Example of sexting: "Hey you! I wanted to share some NSFW ideas with you since you were on my mind. Are you currently into that?

2. Recognize angles

Susan Ruth, a sex educator, and brand strategist advise, "Know your angles if you're including picture or video into your sexting practice." The views that keep you the most technologically secure are what I mean when I say, "I don't mean the view that makes your ass seem like the greatest version of itself. When it comes to sexting, we seldom want to consider sexual and online safety, but you must.

Ruth raises an excellent point. Even if you trust your partner and are sexting with them, you may never be sure where those images will wind up. Do yourself a favor and conceal your tattoos and other distinctive traits when it comes to your face. For fun, you could even add a faux tattoo.

As an illustration of sexting, say, "I'm sending you a snapshot of my hand down my underwear and I want you to know I'm wishing they were your hands instead."

3. Continue to tease

There is no point in hurrying it, just as there is no point in rushing sex. Don't reveal everything in the first sext, Sinclair advises. Send them an explicit photo or tell them what you want to do to them. Give it some time.

Example of sexting: "Imagining what I want to do to you has been making me insane. Every time I contemplate it, I get more and more aroused.

4. Be original

Sexting doesn't have to imply grabbing someone by the genitalia, unlike what some people may believe. Tell me what you would do to me if we were in a room together with nothing but whipped cream, a single candle, and no mattress in sight, like in the sexting scenario above.

5. Continue with the foreplay

When sexting, you shouldn't miss the foreplay if you wouldn't skip it when you're with someone in person. According to Sinclair, "the buildup and foreplay in any sexual activity are what helps make the big finish so spectacular."

For example, Let's take this as far as we can gently, in sexting terms. then let loose with the orgasm.

Chapter 5

Dare Foreplay!

The dance movements that all women like

It's time to move on to seduction, pick one or two of the foreplay techniques from the list below as you please, give them a try, and I nearly promise she'll be pleading for it in no time. This list provides some insight into the foreplay techniques that women adore most.

Just keep in mind that not all women like all types of foreplay, so it's a good idea to have some backup moves prepared in case she doesn't enjoy the ones you've selected, allowing you to move on to something she would enjoy.

1. A kiss

It should almost always be at the top of the list. Women like kissing because it starts everything else in motion. Just be careful not to use too much tongue at first or leave her covered in spittle, otherwise, she could believe she just got come on by an alpaca! Start mild and build up to hard pressure.

2 Nibbling

Women like a little mild nibbling, but you will need to determine where she enjoys it the most. If in doubt, begin at the ears and attempt to travel around her body while alternating between steps 3 and 4. Just be sure it's a little bit and not something she would anticipate coming from a tiger shark.

3.Massage Start with the shoulders or the feet and gradually work your way up to the whole body. Spending some time getting a full body massage is the most reliable method to transition from perhaps innocent intentions to full-blown intense lovemaking since women like the sensation of having their skin touched.

4. Body kissing

Include this in the massage. Just begin by giving the odd peck in between your hand motions, and when the moment is right, completely transition to just using your lips and tongue to continue your cuddling. She'll go crazy for it.

5 All of the aforementioned. Alternate between these four techniques for a time to make her ready for the subsequent, somewhat more intense phases of foreplay.

6 Play the breast

Women often lament the fact that when they are dressed, males spend the whole day staring at their breasts yet do nothing with them in bed. Women's breasts and nipples are often incredibly sensitive, and by stimulating her via them, you have direct access to all other places.

However, you have to develop your intuitive skills to achieve this. Start with kissing, progress to licking, and then attempt a little biting or nibbling as well. Nevertheless, a lot depends on the particular lady. Additionally, keep in mind that while your tongue is working on the nipple, you have two hands that might be softly stroking the whole breast.

7. fingerwork

Possibly the ideal approach is to start by softly massaging and stroking her lower body before moving on to lightly massage the clitoris. Some women like having fingers placed in the vagina, while others dislike it. She'll likely inform you in any direction. Additionally, if this is a course of action you are set on doing, do some research on the technique beforehand since nothing would turn her off more than watching you performing what seemed to be normal plumbing work on her most private areas.

8 Minimal oral

Her favorite segment of the program. But when I say light, I mean just a little bit of mild clitoris and labia stroking with the tip of the tongue. There is currently no penetration.

9. Heavy oral

She'll want something a bit more involved after just a little while of gentle oral, however. Now is the moment to start slapping at her and sometimes piercing her with your tongue. Try softly sucking at the clitoris while flicking your tongue frantically over it, and even try putting fingers in her at the same time, to push her over the edge. If done well, this combo is explosive.

10. Anal stimulation. Unless you are certain that this is what she wants, DON'T TRY IT. Only your intuitive abilities will let you know the truth since many women do like a little mild anal stimulation but won't say it out loud. To observe how she reacts, try inadvertently flicking your tongue over that place now and again while providing oral, just to test the waters.

Chapter 6

Make Love Adventurous

When you can have a great romp, why settle for a good one? We've got the expert-recommended moves that will have her thinking you're a real sex god, from an unexpected position that will get her off to a fresh way to use that pull-up bar.

There are many opportunities for greatness, so there's no reason to settle into a boring routine in bed—even if a night of dull sex is still the most entertaining evening you've had all week. Furthermore, you don't need a special occasion, like Valentine's Day or your birthday, to indulge in some wild behavior in bebed

1 The not-so-lazy boy

Think vertically if you've always had it on the horizontal. Standing sex, according to sex expert Dr. Shetti Lyon, Ph.D., is a tremendous rush that will make you feel like the most macho sex god around—and your partner will concur. There are a few tricks to pulling off this move without breaking a hip, according to Lyon, so it helps if you've been doing your squats. If you need a little extra help, however, for this move you thought only worked in movies, Lyon says there are a few. For balance, lean against a wall or, even better, raise one foot on a cozy chair. Have her wrap her legs around your waist, then watch as your prowess sweeps her off her feet.

2. The O SPOT

Even if you are certain that you are an oral communication expert, the following is something you are likely overlooking: Dr. Pat Putt, Ph.D., a sex psychotherapist explains that the front commissure is a little area just above the clitoris. "It will strike that area if a woman is on top and rubbing up against the pelvic. Additionally, you may apply pressure with the part of your teeth closest to your gums while simultaneously rhythmically stimulating the area with your tongue or a sex object. She could not even be aware of how sensitive she is there, thus it will be a shocking move for her.

3. Showtime

Couples in the same area code don't often consider utilizing video chat to participate in a session of virtual sex, however, long-distance couples may already be on board with this idea. Even if you already reside under the same roof, Putt advises it. Many women have fantasies involving an aspect of voyeurism and exhibitionism, he says. She will either watch you while you watch her touch herself.

4. The so-right angle

If you only descend while she is laying down, consider giving the situation a fresh twist. The following action is advised by the sex coach Lucy Linda: Try asking her to go down on all fours the next time you're ready to have an oral treatment. Laying underneath her on your back with your legs extended out from her body, do oral on her from behind. As opposed to when you're face down, sucking on the clitoris and using your tongue from below feels different, according to Levine. And it allows you to use your tongue to create new erogenous angles.

5. Rough stuff

Kerner advises you to go a step further and add some minor BDSM into the bedroom since you already know your lady has read Fifty Shades of Grey and become a touch flushed with desire. Baby steps are OK if you're unsure if being a bit harsh is truly her (or your) thing.

Chapter 7

Compliment Each Other After Sex

You are fortunate to know someone who can wrap his arms around you and make you feel safe and cherished. Although highly crucial, a relationship should not just be built on a physical connection. To express how much you respect him in your life, you must utilize words. But often, you're correct, those words are hard to come by, particularly when you're not sure what to say after sex.

Here are 20 sultry and seductive things to say after sex to increase closeness and solidify your bond

1 "I'm very fortunate to have you right here with me."

2. "You know just how to cheer me up,"

3. "You're making me swelter."

4. "I've really missed you!"

5. "Baby, you make me crazy."

6. "That was very amazing!"

7. "You have such beautiful eyes; I could gaze at them for hours."

8. "How do you look so hot?"

9. "When you stare at me like that, my heart skips a beat."

10. "How did you learn all of this?"

11. "Nothing compares to curling up next to you."

12. "I definitely needed this today"

13. "You are very fantastic"

14. "I like it when you go into me"

15. "This is like paradise, lying here with you."

16. "I've never been with somebody as incredible as you!"

17. "I really hope it was as beneficial to you as it was to me."

18. "Keep holding me in this position."

19. "I wouldn't alter a single thing about you."

20. "You give me such wonderful feelings."

Chapter 8

Take a Bath Together

After having a passionate love affair, taking a bath together just strengthens the relationship and fosters love and devotion. Have a bath together after sexual activity. You may sneakily enter the bathtub with your husband; who knows, something could begin there. A nice, bubbly bath would be preferable.